Glycemic Index Diet:

Improve Health, Using the Glycemic Index Guide, With Delicious Glycemic Index Recipes

JENNIFER COLLINS

TABLE OF CONTENTS

Introduction: a Glycemic Index Guide

The glycemic index is a method of ranking foods based on how they affect blood sugar levels. It's a scale which is often used by dieticians to demonstrate the impact of consuming certain foods and beverages. Essentially, the glycemic index, or GI, measures how a certain food will affect your blood sugar in comparison to glucose.

Foods which rank higher on the glycemic index are, generally speaking, those which are broken down more quickly by the digestive process, causing a spike in blood sugar levels in a relatively short time frame; these foods are generally those which contain higher levels of refined sugars and other simple carbohydrates. By comparison, foods which rank lower on the glycemic index are digested more slowly and instead result in a more modest increase in blood sugar levels over a longer period of time.

Foods which cause a sudden peak in blood sugar levels contribute to a higher risk of diabetes, heart disease and a variety of other illnesses. These spikes in blood sugar levels can eventually cause you to develop insulin resistance and ultimately, diabetes. By the same token, a diet which is rich in low glycemic index foods helps reduce your risk of diabetes and also makes it far easier to lose weight.

What it all really comes down to is carbohydrates. All carbohydrates are broken down into glucose by the digestive process, but simple carbohydrates, especially refined grain products and refined sugars, are especially problematic. When you hear people talking about a low GI diet, what they're referring to is a diet which greatly reduces and in some cases, completely eliminates foods which are high on the glycemic index. These foods are generally substituted with lower GI alternatives (whole grains like brown rice instead of white rice and whole wheat flour instead of white flour, for instance).

Whether or not you choose to take your diet to this extreme is a choice that you'll need to make for yourself with the advice of your physician. If you're just trying to lose weight rather than going on a low GI diet at the recommendation of your doctor, you'll need to decide for yourself how often – or if – you'll go a little off of your diet for a higher-GI treat.

The glycemic index scale ranks foods from 1 to 100 (with 100 being pure glucose). There are three broad categories to keep in mind if you're trying to watch the GI value of your diet. There are what are considered high GI foods, which rank at 70 or greater on the index, medium GI foods, ranking between 56 and 69 on the index and low GI foods; these are foods which rank at 55 or lower on the index.

Examples of high GI foods include white bread, white rice, glucose (obviously), maltose and some starchy vegetables like potatoes (but not sweet potatoes) and parsnips.

Medium GI foods include some of the starchier fruits (like bananas), partially refined grain products (like many mass produced wheat breads which are not specifically labeled as whole wheat) and ice cream, among others. Beer is generally also classified in the medium GI category, although this may vary depending on the particular style of beer.

Low GI foods are largely complex carbohydrates (the good kind) – whole grains, most vegetables and fruits, beans, nuts and certain natural sweeteners like fructose. Most wines and distilled spirits fall into this category as well, although obviously, it is highly recommended to consume in moderation.

Why Choose a Low GI Diet?

Other than the obvious health benefits such as a lower risk of developing heart disease and insulin resistance leading to diabetes, there is a lot of evidence that it's easier to lose excess weight and maintain a healthy weight on a diet which consists chiefly of low glycemic index foods. This is due to the fact that the average person's energy expenditure is higher when eating a low GI diet – even after they lose excess weight. Their energy expenditure is also higher than that of people who eat a low fat diet which is not designed with the glycemic index in mind. There is still research going on into this area, but the results thus far seem to bear out what proponents of the diet have said for some time now.

A low GI diet offers many benefits, but like any other diet, it's not a panacea. You still need to exercise common sense in terms of portion sizes and to make physical activity a regular part of your life. The American Diabetes Association endorses the diet to a certain extent, but notes that beyond the GI value of foods, people need to be mindful of the total amount of carbohydrates in their diet and use their own judgment about what and how they eat along with other lifestyle factors which affect their health.

Eating a low GI diet doesn't have to mean completely eliminating all of the foods you're used to having, but some may need to be replaced with alternatives which have a less drastic effect on your blood sugar levels. White bread is largely out, however, as is white rice, sugar-laden breakfast cereals made with refined grains (and refined sugars) and sweetened soft drinks. These are foods which really should be avoided, except perhaps as rare treats, whether you're on a low GI diet or simply concerned about your health in general. Instead, try having whole wheat bread or brown rice, oatmeal or seltzer.

A low GI diet isn't just about weight loss, although you certainly can lose weight by eating this kind of diet. It's about feeling better and living a healthier and more than likely, longer life. It's a diet which isn't meant to be a one week crash diet, but a long term (even lifelong) change in lifestyle which can greatly reduce your risk of developing many of the most common diseases in the industrialized world, improve your health and give you more energy due to avoiding the blood sugar roller coaster of a high GI diet. You'll probably lose those extra pounds you've been carrying in the bargain, which is a nice side benefit, no matter how you slice it.

Two quick notes about the recipes in this book are in order. Here and there in the book you will find ingredients listed in recipes which are somewhat higher on the glycemic index; they're used in fairly small amounts and of course, you shouldn't be eating any single recipe three meals per day. At the same time, you should feel free to make appropriate substitutions where necessary in order to adjust them for your own particular requirements.

You'll also note that the dessert section of this book consists of just one recipe. This isn't a mistake. There are of course low GI dessert recipes out there, but desserts have been largely omitted from this particular book for two reasons: skipping dessert (or having a piece of fruit for dessert) is never a bad idea. Additionally, the vast majority of dessert recipes can be made relatively low GI through some very simple adjustments such as using sugar substitutes rather than refined sugars and where possible, whole grains instead of white flour.

In other words, if you can cook enough to use a recipe, you can probably handle reworking existing dessert recipes for a low GI diet easily enough. No one cookbook can give you every possible recipe; but after you've tried a few of the recipes which follow, you'll be excited about cooking low GI dishes and ready to do some exploring of your own – think of this book as your launch pad to healthy culinary exploration. Without further ado, let's get to the recipes!

Lunch and Dinner Entrees

Fish Casserole

Number of servings: 4

Ingredients

1 lb white fish (cod, sole, haddock or any other you like), cut into
2" pieces
6 medium sized potatoes, cubed
1 medium sized carrot, sliced
1 medium sized onion, diced
4 cloves of garlic, sliced

Juice of 1 lemon

2 tbsp chopped parsley
salt and black pepper, to taste
a large pinch of dill
1 tbsp olive oil

Preparation:

Start by preheating your oven to 375 F and oil a large (9" x 13")
baking dish. Place the fish in the baking dish and drizzle with
lemon juice. Add the vegetables and parsley and stir gently to
combine. Sprinkle with the dill, salt and black pepper to taste.
Cover the dish and bake for 1 hour.

Turkey Meatloaf

Number of servings: 8 – 10

Ingredients:

2 lbs lean ground turkey
1 medium sized yellow onion, diced
2 cloves of garlic, minced
1 stalk of celery, diced
1 cup tomato sauce or pureed tomato (use reduced sugar or sugar free tomato sauce)
½ cup finely chopped Italian flat leaf parsley
2 tbsp reduced sugar catsup
2 tbsp Dijon mustard
2 large eggs
1 tbsp oregano
1tbsp olive oil
salt and black pepper, to taste

Preparation:

Preheat your oven to 350 while you heat the olive oil in a skillet over medium heat. Once the oil is hot, add the celery, garlic and onion and sauté until they turn translucent, about 3 minutes, stirring occasionally. Remove from heat and transfer to a large bowl with the ground turkey, eggs, oregano, mustard, catsup, parsley and some salt and black pepper. Mix well to thoroughly combine, using your hands to mix.

Transfer the mixture to a large (9" x 13") baking dish or divide and bake in two smaller dishes. Pour the tomato sauce over the top of the meatloaf, cover with foil and bake for 1 hour – if you like your meatloaf slightly crisped on top, remove the foil about 40 minutes into baking. When the meatloaf is done, remove from the oven and allow to rest for about 5 minutes before slicing and serving.

Cauliflower and Chickpea Curry

Number of servings: 6

Ingredients:

1 ½ cups cooked chickpeas (about 1 can if using canned chickpeas), drained and rinsed
1 large or 2 medium sized heads of cauliflower, minced or shredded with a grater
1 large yellow onion, diced small
1 Thai chili, minced (may use more or less to taste)
4 cloves of garlic, minced
3 tbsp canola or vegetable oil (not olive oil)
1 tbsp garam masala (curry powder may be substituted, if desired)
2 tsp powdered turmeric
2 tsp ground coriander
1 tsp cumin seeds
1 tsp mustard seeds
1 tsp methi*
salt and black pepper, to taste

* methi is dried fenugreek leaves; you can find this spice at Indian, Pakistani and Bangladeshi groceries and some health food stores – simply omit this ingredient if you can't find it, since there's really no substitute.

Preparation:

Heat the oil over medium heat in a large, heavy skillet. Once the oil is hot, add the mustard seeds and cook until they start to pop, 30 seconds to 1 minute. Add the cumin seeds and cook for another 30 seconds or until they become fragrant. Add the onion and garlic and cook until golden brown (about 7 – 8 minutes), stirring regularly. Add the coriander, garam masala or curry powder and turmeric, along with just a little salt and black pepper and cook, stirring regularly for another 1 - 2 minutes, then reduce the heat to medium – low.

Add the cauliflower and chickpeas and cook for about 10 minutes, or until the cauliflower is tender and the chickpeas are heated through, stirring occasionally. Remove from heat, season to taste with salt and black pepper and serve hot with brown rice or whole wheat naan.

Stuffed Shells

Number of servings: 6

Ingredients:

6 ounces large pasta shells
½ cup sliced crimini mushrooms
½ cup chopped spinach
½ cup chopped Italian flat leaf parsley
1 cup tomato sauce (homemade or premade sugar-free sauce)
1 cup low fat ricotta cheese
½ cup low fat parmesan or Romano cheese
3 cloves of garlic, minced
1 egg
1 tbsp olive oil
1 tsp oregano
1 tsp basil
salt and black pepper, to taste

Preparation:

Start by preheating your oven to 375 F. Cook the pasta until al dente, drain, rinse in cold water and reserve. Heat the olive oil in a skillet over medium heat; once the oil is hot, add the garlic and mushrooms. Cook for about 5 minutes, or until the mushrooms and garlic are tender and start to turn golden brown. Remove from heat and transfer the sautéed garlic and mushrooms to a large bowl.

Add the spinach to the skillet and cook until wilted; remove from heat and transfer to the bowl along with the mushrooms. Add the egg, cheeses and spices to a small saucepan over medium – low heat until the cheeses melt together. Pour the cheese mixture into the spinach and mushroom mixture, stir well to combine and season to taste with salt and black pepper.

Fill the shells with the cheese and vegetable mixture and place in a large baking dish. Pour the tomato sauce over the shells and bake for 25 minutes. Remove from the oven and serve hot.

Citrus – Mustard Chicken

Number of servings: 4

Ingredients:

4 chicken breasts, boneless and skinless, cut into bite sized pieces
½ cup Dijon mustard
1 tbsp olive oil
Juice of 1 lemon
juice of 1 lime
salt and black pepper, to taste

Preparation:

Heat the olive oil over medium heat in a large skillet. Once the oil is hot, add the chicken and cook until lightly browned, turning every few minutes to ensure that all sides are evenly browned. Add the lemon and lime juice and the mustard and stir to combine. Reduce the heat to medium low and cook for about 10 minutes or until the chicken pieces are cooked through, stirring occasionally. Remove from heat and serve immediately.

Curried Winter Vegetable and Lentil Casserole

Number of servings: 4

Ingredients:

2 large parsnips, scrubbed, trimmed and sliced into ½" pieces*
4 medium sized carrots, scrubbed, trimmed and sliced into ½" pieces
1 large potato, scrubbed and cubed
1 large sweet potato, scrubbed and cubed
1 large onion, diced
4 cloves of garlic, chopped
3 ½ cups vegetable broth
½ cup dry red lentils
2 tbsp red curry paste (or any other type you prefer)
2 tbsp vegetable oil
2 tbsp cilantro, chopped
salt and black pepper, to taste

* This ingredient may be omitted or substituted with a lower GI vegetable; parsnips are fairly high on the glycemic index, so if you're in doubt, simply omit them.

Preparation:

Heat the vegetable oil in a large saucepan over medium heat; once the oil is hot, add the garlic and onion and cook for about 3 minutes, or until tender. Add the potatoes, parsnips and carrots, then increase the heat to medium – high and cook until the vegetables are lightly browned, about 7 – 8 minutes.

Add the vegetable broth and curry paste, stir well to combine and bring the mixture to a boil, then reduce the heat to a simmer and add the lentils. Cover and cook for about 15 minutes or until the lentils are tender and the mixture is thickened. Preheat your oven to 400 F, remove the pot from heat and season to taste with salt and black pepper.

Transfer the mixture to a large (9" x 13") baking dish. Sprinkle the casserole with chopped cilantro and transfer to the oven. Bake for 20 minutes, or until the casserole is lightly browned. Remove the casserole from the oven and serve hot.

Barley and Pea Risotto

Number of servings: 4

Ingredients:

1 ½ cups dry barley
7 cups vegetable stock
1 cup dry white wine
1 small onion, minced
3 cloves of garlic, minced
1 cup peas (fresh or frozen)
a handful of fresh chives (1 -2 bunches), chopped
2 tbsp olive oil
2 tbsp grated Romano or Parmesan cheese
salt and black pepper, to taste

Preparation:

Heat the olive oil in a large saucepan over medium heat. Once the oil is hot, add the garlic and onion and sauté until fragrant, about 2 minutes, stirring occasionally. Add the barley and cook for another 2 – 3 minutes, stirring regularly.

Add the wine and 1 cup of the vegetable stock. Simmer, stirring regularly and add more vegetable stock a little at a time as the barley absorbs the stock; this should take about 20 minutes. Once most of the liquid has been absorbed, add the peas and stir in. Cook for another 5 minutes, or until all of the liquid has been absorbed and the peas are heated through. Stir in the Romano or Parmesan and all but a little bit of the chives. Remove from heat, season to taste with salt and black pepper and stir again. Serve hot topped with a sprinkling of chives.

German-Style Roast Pork (or Lamb)

Number of servings: 4

Ingredients:

4 lean pork (or lamb) tenderloin medallions, about 4 ounces each
12 crimini or button mushrooms, washed and sliced thinly
1 red onion, sliced
1 cup sauerkraut
1 cup water
1 tsp caraway seeds
6 juniper berries (optional)
salt and black pepper, to taste

Preparation:

Start by preheating your oven to 350 F. While the oven is heating up, place the pork in a baking dish and top with the mushrooms, followed by the sauerkraut and then the sliced onion. Add the water to the baking dish, along with the juniper berries (if using). Sprinkle the pork with caraway seeds and a little black pepper, then bake for about 35 minutes or until the pork is cooked through, basting once with the cooking liquid halfway through. Once the pork is done, remove the dish from the oven and serve at once. Discard the juniper berries before serving, if you used them in this dish.

Trinidadian-Style Stuffed Sweet Potatoes

Number of servings: 4 2x ingredients

Ingredients:

4 sweet potatoes, scrubbed
1 large yellow onion, diced
4 cloves of garlic, minced
2 cups cooked chickpeas, drained and rinsed if using canned
2 tbsp hot curry powder (use Caribbean curry powder if possible)
¼ cup finely chopped cilantro
½ of a habanero pepper, seeded and minced, or more to taste (optional)
2 tsp white wine vinegar
2 tsp vegetable oil
2 tsp dried thyme
salt and black pepper, to taste

Preparation:

Preheat your oven to 400 F. Pierce each sweet potato a few times with a fork or knife and place on a foil-lined baking sheet. Bake the sweet potatoes for about 45 minutes or until tender. Remove from the oven and set aside.

While the sweet potatoes are baking, you can prepare the filling. Heat the vegetable oil in a saucepan over medium heat. Add the garlic, onion, cilantro and habanero (if using) and sauté until the garlic and onion start to become tender and the cilantro is completely wilted, about 3 – 4 minutes, stirring occasionally. Add the thyme, curry powder, chickpeas and vinegar and stir well to combine. Cook until heated through, remove from heat, cover and set aside.

Once the sweet potatoes are cool enough to handle safely, slice them open and scoop out most of the flesh, transferring it to the pan with the chickpea mixture. Reserve the sweet potato skins.

Cook the chickpea and sweet potato mixture over medium heat until heated through; season to taste with salt and black pepper and divide the mixture among the sweet potato skins and return them to the oven. Bake the stuffed sweet potatoes for about 20 minutes, or until the filling is slightly browned on top. Remove from the oven and serve immediately with hot pepper sauce on the side.

North African Style Spaghetti with Vegetables

Number of servings: 4

Ingredients:

12 ounces whole wheat spaghetti or fettucine (about ¾ of a
standard 16 ounce package)
2 ½ cups diced tomatoes
1 cup cooked red kidney beans (drained and rinsed, if using canned
kidney beans)
4 cloves of garlic, minced
10 crimini mushrooms, washed and sliced
1 red onion, diced small
1 cup chopped Italian parsley
½ cup chopped cilantro
2 tsp cumin
2 tsp turmeric
a pinch of cinnamon
a pinch of cayenne pepper
salt and black pepper, to taste
cooking spray

Preparation:

Cook the spaghetti or fettuccine according to the directions on the
package. While the pasta cooks, spray a large skillet with cooking
spray and heat over medium heat. When the skillet is hot, sauté the
mushrooms, onion and garlic until soft, about 5 minutes, stirring
regularly.

Add the diced tomato and spices and cook for 5 – 7 minutes or
until the tomatoes soften, stirring regularly. Add the kidney beans
and cook for a few minutes until the beans are heated through. Add
the parsley and cilantro and cook until just wilted. By now the
pasta should be cooked and drained, so add it to the skillet and stir
to combine with the other ingredients. Remove from heat and serve
at once.

Imam Bayaldi (Turkish Style Stuffed Eggplant)

Number of servings: 4

Ingredients:

2 large eggplants (about 1 lb each)
1 lb lean ground turkey
1 small white or red onion, diced small
1 tomato, diced
1 red bell pepper, diced
1 bunch of parsley, chopped
4 cloves of garlic, minced
2 tbsp olive oil
2 tbsp finely crumbled feta cheese
1 tsp oregano
salt and black pepper, to taste
cooking spray

Preparation:

Start by preheating your oven to 400 F. Pierce the eggplants in a few places with a fork or a sharp knife and place on a baking sheet lightly coated with cooking spray. Roast the eggplants for about 30 minutes or until they collapse. Remove from the oven and set aside until they're cool enough to handle. Cut the eggplants in half lengthwise and scoop out the flesh, leaving about ¼ inch of flesh inside; reserve the skins. Chop the cooked eggplant flesh into bite sized pieces and set aside.

Heat half of the olive oil in a skillet over medium heat. Once the oil is hot, add the diced bell pepper and onion and cook until tender (about 6 – 7 minutes), stirring occasionally. Add the ground turkey and garlic and cook, stirring constantly to break up the turkey until thoroughly browned, 5 – 6 minutes. Return the chopped eggplant to the skillet, along with the parsley, diced tomato and oregano. Reduce the heat to medium low and cook for 10 – 15 minutes, or until thickened, stirring regularly. Remove from heat and season to taste with salt and black pepper.

Add a little more cooking spray to the baking sheet, then transfer the reserved eggplant skins to the prepared baking sheet. Divide the turkey and vegetable mixture among the eggplant skins, then drizzle with the remaining olive oil and sprinkle with the crumbled feta. Bake for 15 minutes or until the eggplant is heated through and the tips are lightly browned. Remove from heat and serve at once.

Parmesan – Herb Crusted Salmon

Number of servings: 4

Ingredients:

4 salmon filets, about 4 ounces each
1 cup whole wheat bread crumbs (premade or make your own)
½ cup grated Romano or Parmesan cheese
2 tbsp chopped Italian parsley
1 tbsp olive oil
Juice of ½ lime
black pepper, to taste
cooking spray

Preparation:

Preheat your oven to 400 F. Add the bread crumbs, parsley, Parmesan, olive oil and lime juice to a blender or food processor and blend until thoroughly combined; transfer to a large plate. Season the salmon filets with black pepper and coat with the bread crumb mixture.

Lightly coat a baking sheet with cooking spray. Place the salmon filets on the prepared baking sheet and bake for about 10 minutes, or until they turn golden brown and the salmon is cooked through. Remove the salmon filets from the oven and serve immediately.

Mexican-Style Low GI Vegetarian Chili

Number of servings: 4

Ingredients:

1 ½ cup cooked kidney beans (or 1 can, drained and rinsed)
1 cup sliced mushrooms (crimini or button, your choice)
1 ½ cups diced tomatoes, preferably fresh, but canned may be substituted
1 cup diced zucchini
½ cup corn kernels (fresh or frozen, don't use canned corn)
1 large yellow onion, diced
4 cloves of garlic, minced
1 – 2 jalapeno or Serrano peppers, or to taste
2 tbsp unsweetened cocoa powder
2 tbsp chopped cilantro
1 tbsp red wine vinegar
1 tbsp olive oil or vegetable oil
2 tsp dried oregano or 2 tbsp fresh oregano leaves, minced
salt and black pepper, to taste

Preparation:

Heat the olive oil in a large saucepan over medium heat; once the oil is hot, add the onion and garlic and cook until they start to turn translucent, about 3 – 4 minutes, stirring occasionally. Add the oregano, zucchini and peppers and continue cooking for another 3 minutes. Add the remaining ingredients and stir well to combine. Cover the pan and simmer, covered, for 35 minutes over medium – low heat. Remove from heat, season to taste with salt and black pepper and serve hot.

Beef Stroganoff

Number of servings: 12

Ingredients:

2 lbs lean ground beef
1 large yellow onion, diced
1 bulb of garlic, chopped (but not minced)
2 cups beef stock
2 cups of sliced crimini mushrooms (or 1 cup each crimini and button mushrooms)
2 cups lowfat plain yogurt
1 cup dry red wine
½ cup flour (use whole wheat if possible)
¼ cup finely chopped Italian flat leaf parsley
2 tbsp olive oil
2 tsp paprika
salt and black pepper, to taste

Preparation:

Heat the olive oil in a large, heavy skillet over medium heat; once the oil is hot, add the onions, garlic and mushrooms and sauté until tender. Add the beef, parsley, paprika, a little salt and a lot of black pepper and continue cooking until the beef is browned, stirring regularly to break up the meat into smaller pieces. Stir in the flour and continue cooking for 2 minutes, stirring occasionally. Pour in the wine and beef stock and continue cooking until the sauce thickens and is slightly reduced. Add the yogurt and stir until the sauce is smooth. Remove from heat and serve hot over whole grain noodles.

Pork (or Lamb) Tenderloin with French Onion Sauce

Number of servings: 4

Ingredients:

16 ounces pork (or better -- lamb) tenderloin, trimmed of fat and sliced into bite sized pieces
2 medium sized yellow onions, sliced thinly
1 green bell pepper, seeded and sliced into thin strips
3 cloves of garlic, minced
2 cups beef stock
1 tbsp vegetable oil
1 tsp dried rosemary (or 2 ½ tsp fresh, finely chopped rosemary)
salt and black pepper, to taste

Preparation:

Season the pork pieces with a little salt, black pepper and rosemary while you heat ½ tbsp of vegetable oil in a large skillet over medium heat. Add the pork to the skillet and brown, turning to brown all sides. Remove the pork from the skillet and set aside.

Add the onions, garlic and green pepper slices to the skillet and cook for about 6 minutes or until the onions and garlic start to turn golden brown, stirring occasionally. Add the beef stock and a little more salt and pepper to the skillet and bring the mixture to a boil; boil until the stock is reduced to about ¾ cup (a little more than half).

Reduce the heat to medium high, return the pork to the skillet and cook for another 3 – 4 minutes, or until the pork is thoroughly cooked through, stirring occasionally. Remove from heat and serve immediately, drizzled with the remaining sauce.

Chile Relleno Casserole

Number of servings: 8

Ingredients:

8 large poblano chilies, roasted, peeled and seeded*
1 ½ cup reduced fat shredded cheese (Monterey Jack is a good choice, but use whatever you like)

3 eggs
½ cup half and half
2 tsp oregano
2 tbsp finely chopped cilantro
salt and black pepper, to taste
salsa, for serving (your choice)
cooking spray

* This can be done ahead of time. You can roast the poblanos under your oven's broiler or over the flame of a gas stove, turning occasionally until the skins start to blister and blacken. Place the roasted peppers in a paper bag and fold shut to seal. Set the peppers aside for about 10 minutes; they'll steam in the bag, which will make them much easier to peel. Rub the peppers under cold running water; the skins will come off easily. Chop off the tops of the peppers, slice open and remove the seeds, then set them aside until you're ready to prepare your casserole.

Preparation:

Preheat your oven to 350 F and lightly coat an 8" x 8" baking dish with cooking spray. Lay half of your prepared Poblanos in the bottom of the dish to form a single layer. Sprinkle half of the cheese over the chilies, then top with the rest of the Poblanos. Whisk together the eggs, cilantro, half and half and a little salt and black pepper and pour the mixture over the chilies, followed by the rest of the cheese. Bake, uncovered, for about 35 minutes or until the cheese is bubbling and golden brown. Remove from the oven and allow to rest for 10 minutes before serving with the salsa of your choice.

Pasta with Scallops

Number of servings: 6

Ingredients:

8 ounces whole wheat fettuccine or spaghetti (1/2 of a package)
1 lb fresh scallops (or frozen and thawed)
1 red onion, sliced thinly
2 cloves of garlic, minced
1 ½ cups sliced crimini or button mushrooms
1/2 cup olive oil
2 tsp vegetable oil (or olive oil)
¼ cup red wine vinegar
1 tsp basil

salt and black pepper, to taste
a little chopped parsley (about 2 tbsp), for serving

Preparation:

Cook the pasta according to the directions on the package (try to get it at al dente consistency). Drain and set aside, covered to keep warm. Heat the oil over medium heat in a large skillet. Add the garlic, onion and mushroom and cook until the onions begin to become tender, about 3 minutes, stirring occasionally. Add the scallops and continue cooking for another 3 – 4 minutes, or until the scallops are opaque, stirring regularly. Remove from heat and whisk together the olive oil, vinegar, oregano and a little salt and black pepper. Add the pasta to the skillet, pour in the vinaigrette and toss to combine. Serve immediately, topped with a little chopped parsley.

Low GI Chicken Salad

Number of servings: 8

Ingredients:

2 lbs chicken breasts, boneless, skinless and trimmed of fat
1 cup plain yogurt
1 cup grapes (red or green, your choice), halved
1 stalk of celery, diced small
1/2 of a small red onion, diced small
salt, black pepper, to taste

Preparation:

Cook the chicken any way you like (boiled, roasted, grilled – just make sure it's cooked through). Allow the chicken to cool until it's safe to handle; while it cools, you can prepare the onion, celery and grapes. Shred the chicken with a fork and transfer to a large bowl. Add the remaining ingredients, stir well to combine and season to taste with salt and black pepper. Cover and refrigerate for at least 1 hour and serve cold on lettuce leaves or as sandwiches.

Low GI Tortilla Crust Pizza

Number of servings: 4

Ingredients:

4 whole wheat tortillas
1 cup shredded low fat mozzarella cheese
1 cup sliced mushrooms
1 cup sliced black olives
1 cup baby spinach
2 cloves of garlic, minced
4 tbsp tomato sauce (sugar free, homemade or premade)
1 tbsp olive oil, plus a little extra for brushing the tortillas

Preparation:

Preheat your oven to 400 F. Heat the olive oil in a large skillet; once the oil is hot, add the garlic, mushrooms and spinach and saute until the mushrooms are soft and the spinach wilts, about 3 minutes, stirring occasionally. Remove from heat and set aside. Brush the tortillas with a little bit of olive oil, place on a large baking sheet and spread each with a portion of the tomato sauce. Divide the mushroom and spinach mixture among the tortillas and sprinkle each with ¼ cup of the shredded mozzarella. Bake for 10 – 12 minutes, or until the cheese bubbles and turns golden brown. Remove from the oven and serve hot.

Sausage and Pumpkin Soup

Number of servings: 6 – 8

Ingredients:

1 lb Italian sausage (sweet or hot, your choice)
1 medium sized yellow onion, diced small
4 cups chicken or vegetable stock
1 ½ cups sliced mushrooms (crimini or button)
1 ½ cups pureed pumpkin (or 1 15 ounce can)
4 cloves of garlic, minced
½ cup plain yogurt
½ cup milk
½ cup water
2 tsp olive oil
1 tsp oregano
1 tsp basil
salt, black pepper and crushed red pepper, to taste

Preparation:

Heat the olive oil in a large skillet over medium heat. Once the oil
is hot, add the sausage and cook until cooked through and
browned, breaking the sausage into pieces as you go. Drain off
excess fat and add the garlic, onion, spices and mushrooms and
cook until the mushrooms are tender, about 5 minutes, stirring
occasionally. Add the stock and pumpkin and stir well to combine.
Bring to a boil, then reduce the heat to medium low and simmer for
30 minutes, stirring occasionally. Remove from heat, add the milk,
yogurt, water and salt, black pepper and crushed red pepper flakes
to taste. Serve hot.

Stuffed Chicken Breasts

Number of servings: 6

Ingredients:

3 chicken breasts, halved lengthwise
1 ½ cups finely chopped broccoli
1/3 cup bread crumbs
2 cloves of garlic, minced
1 egg
4 ounces cream cheese, softened at room temperature
2 tbsp grated Parmesan or Romano cheese
salt and black pepper, to taste
cooking spray

Preparation:

Start by preheating your oven to 400 F. Spread the inside of each of the halved chicken breasts with a portion of the cream cheese and set aside. Mix the remaining ingredients together in a bowl, stirring well to combine and stuff each chicken breast with the broccoli mixture. Lightly coat a large baking dish with cooking spray, place the chicken breasts into the dish and bake for about 30 minutes or until the chicken is cooked through.

Beef and Vegetable Stir Fry

Number of servings: 4

Ingredients:

1 lb beef sirloin, trimmed and cut into 1" cubes
2 green bell peppers, cubed
1 red onion, diced
½ cup beef stock
¼ cup low sodium soy sauce or tamari
1 tbsp minced ginger
1 tbsp vegetable oil
2 cloves of garlic, minced
juice of 1 lime
black pepper and crushed red pepper flakes, to taste

Preparation:

Add the cubed beef, garlic, ginger and lime juice to a non-reactive (glass or plastic) bowl, along with a little black pepper and crushed red pepper flakes. Toss well to coat and allow the beef to marinate for at least 30 minutes at room temperature. Heat the vegetable oil in a large skillet over medium heat; once the oil is hot, add the beef and brown, turning occasionally to brown all sides evenly, 5- 7 minutes. Add the bell peppers and onions and cook until crisp-tender, stirring occasionally. Serve hot over brown rice or whole wheat noodles.

Beef Stew

Number of servings: 6 – 8

Ingredients:

1 lb lean beef stew meat
2 large yellow onions, diced
4 parsnips, cut into 1" slices
4 large carrots, cut into 1" slices
5 medium sized potatoes, scrubbed and cubed
6 cloves of garlic, minced
2 cups of water
2 cups of beef stock
2 tbsp whole wheat flour
1 tbsp oregano
1 tbsp olive oil
1 tbsp red wine vinegar
½ tsp dill
½ tsp paprika
1 bay leaf
salt and black pepper, to taste

Preparation:

Heat the olive oil in a large skillet over medium heat; once the oil is hot, add the garlic and onion and sauté until they start to turn translucent, 3 – 4 minutes, stirring occasionally. Add the stew meat to the pot and brown, turning occasionally to cook all sides evenly. Transfer the meat, garlic and onion to a stock pot. Add the remaining ingredients to the pot, bring to a boil and then reduce the heat to medium low and cover. Simmer, covered, for 1 to 2 hours. Season to taste with salt and black pepper and serve hot.

Turkey and Cheese Burritos

Number of servings: 2 (double it)

Ingredients:

2 large (burrito size) whole wheat tortillas
½ lb lean ground turkey
½ of a small red onion, diced
½ cup shredded sharp cheddar cheese
1 tbsp plain Greek yogurt
1 tbsp chopped cilantro
1 tsp cumin
salt and black pepper, to taste
salsa (your choice), to taste
2 tsp olive oil, for browning the turkey

Preparation:

Heat the olive oil in a large skillet over medium heat; add the turkey and half of the diced onion and cook until well browned, stirring regularly to break up the meat into small pieces. Drain and place in a medium sized bowl. Combine with the cilantro, cumin and salt and black pepper to taste. Divide the turkey mixture between two warmed tortillas, top with cheese, Greek yogurt, diced onion and salsa and fold up into burritos. Serve at once with additional salsa on the side.

Stuffed Peppers

Number of servings: 4

Ingredients:

4 large green bell peppers
4 large tomatoes, diced
2 cups cooked brown rice
1 medium sized yellow onion
1 stalk of celery, diced
1 cup sliced mushrooms
6 cloves of garlic, minced
2 eggs, beaten
4 tbsp shredded mozzarella cheese
2 tsp basil
2 tsp thyme
cooking spray

Preparation:

Start by preheating your oven to 350 and bringing a large pot of water to a boil. Slice off the tops of the peppers and remove the seeds and ribs. Once the water is boiling, add the peppers and boil for about 2 minutes – remove the peppers from the boiling water and place in a bowl of cold water. Set aside and heat a large skillet coated with cooking spray over medium heat. Add the onion, garlic, celery and mushrooms and sauté until the vegetables are tender, about 3 – 4 minutes, stirring occasionally. Add the mushrooms and continue cooking until the tomatoes begin to break down into a sauce, about 7 minutes, stirring regularly. Remove from heat and transfer to a large bowl. Add the rice, spices and stir well to combine. Stuff the peppers with the rice and vegetable mixture, place in a 8" x 8" baking dish and bake, covered with foil, for 45 minutes. Remove the foil, top each stuffed pepper with shredded mozzarella and bake for another 15 minutes, or until the cheese bubbles and is very slightly browned. Remove the peppers from the oven and allow them to rest for 5 – 10 minutes before serving.

Side Dishes, Soups and Snacks

Spinach – Artichoke Dip

Number of servings: 8

Ingredients:

1 ½ cups cooked spinach, drained well and cooled to room temperature
1 cup artichoke hearts (from a jar), drained and chopped finely
½ cup cream cheese, softened at room temperature
½ cup water chestnuts, drained and diced small
¼ cup mayonnaise
¼ cup plain Greek yogurt
2 cloves of garlic
2 tbsp minced shallot
1 tsp olive oil
salt, black pepper and cayenne pepper, to taste

Preparation:

Mix the mayonnaise, cream cheese and yogurt in a large bowl. Add a little black pepper and cayenne pepper and stir to incorporate. Add the artichoke hearts, spinach, garlic and shallots, water chestnuts and a little more black pepper and cayenne, if desired. Taste and adjust the seasonings as needed. Refrigerate and serve cold.

Stuffed Mushrooms

Number of servings: 10

Ingredients:

24 crimini mushrooms, washed, patted dry, stems removed
½ of a small yellow onion
2 cups spinach, wilted and chopped finely

2 tbsp minced red bell pepper
2 cloves of garlic, minced
2 tbsp seasoned bread crumbs
1 tbsp finely chopped Italian parsley
1 egg, beaten
½ cup grated Romano or Parmesan cheese
black pepper, to taste

Preparation:

Start by preheating your oven to 400 F. Mix together all of the ingredients except for the mushroom caps in a bowl. Stuff the mushroom caps with the mixture and place on a large non-stick baking sheet; bake for 20 minutes or until the tops are lightly browned and the mushrooms are tender. Remove from the oven and allow to cool slightly before serving or allow them to cool completely and serve at room temperature.

Broccoli with Garlic and Cranberries

Number of servings: 4

Ingredients:

2 large heads of broccoli, cut into bite sized florets (about 4 cups)
4 cloves of garlic, minced (or more to taste)
1 tbsp olive oil
½ cup craisins
salt and black pepper, to taste

Preparation:

Heat the oil over medium heat in a large skillet. Once the oil is hot, add the garlic and sauté until fragrant. Add the broccoli and craisins and sauté until the broccoli is slightly tender but still crisp, 3 – 5 minutes. Remove from heat, season to taste with salt and black pepper and serve hot.

Tabbouleh

Number of servings: 4

Ingredients:

2 cups water
1 cup bulgur wheat
2 cloves of garlic, minced
½ of a small cucumber, diced
2 Roma tomatoes, diced
juice of 1 lemon
zest of ½ lemon
1 cup finely chopped Italian parsley
¼ cup chopped fresh mint
2 tbsp olive oil (use extra virgin olive oil, if you have it on hand)
salt and black pepper, to taste

Preparation:

Bring 2 cups water to a boil; once the water is boiling, add the bulgur, reduce the heat to low and cover. Cook the bulgur for 10 - 12 minutes, or until the water has been absorbed and the bulgur is tender. Transfer the cooked bulgur to a large bowl and set aside to cool.

Add the olive oil, lemon juice and zest to a small bowl and whisk to combine. Pour the dressing over the bulgur and stir. Add the diced tomato, cucumber, parsley and mint and stir to combine. Season to taste with salt and black pepper, stir and refrigerate. Serve cold or at room temperature, if desired.

Easy Brussels Sprouts

Number of servings: 4

Ingredients:

1 lb Brussels sprouts, washed, trimmed and halved
2 – 3 cloves of garlic, minced
½ of a shallot, minced
½ cup vegetable broth
1 tbsp olive or vegetable oil
salt, black pepper and crushed red pepper flakes, to taste
a splash of red wine vinegar (optional)

1 pound fresh brussels sprouts, halved

Preparation:

Heat the oil in a saucepan over medium heat. Add the minced shallots and garlic and cook for about 2 minutes, or until they become fragrant and start to become tender, stirring occasionally.

Add the Brussels sprouts and cook for another 5 minutes, or until they're slightly browned on the outside. Pour the vegetable broth over the Brussels sprouts and increase the heat to medium high. Continue cooking until the broth has almost entirely boiled off. Remove from heat and season to taste with salt, black pepper and crushed red pepper flakes and serve hot.

Collard Greens

Number of servings: 4

Ingredients:

2 large bunches of collard greens, trimmed, washed, patted dry and sliced into ½" ribbons
2 cups vegetable or chicken stock
4 cloves of garlic, minced or crushed
½ of a small red onion, minced
1 Roma tomato, diced small
¼ cup (about 2 ounces) smoked turkey breast, diced small
1 tbsp olive oil
salt, black pepper and crushed red pepper, to taste

Preparation:

Add the olive oil to a large saucepan or stock pot over medium heat. Once the oil is hot, add the garlic and onion and sauté, stirring occasionally, until the garlic and onion are golden brown, about 5 – 7 minutes. Add the vegetable or chicken stock and the diced smoked turkey. Cover and allow the mixture to simmer for about 10 minutes to infuse the stock with the flavor of the other ingredients.

Add the collard greens and increase the heat to medium – high. Cover the pot and cook, covered for 15 minutes, then stir, cover and cook for another 10 minutes, or until the collards are just tender. Remove from heat, season to taste with salt, black pepper and crushed red pepper flakes and serve hot, topped with a spoonful of the cooking liquid.

White Bean Soup

Number of servings: 6

Ingredients:

¾ lb dry white beans (navy, cannellini, great northern, etc.), soaked for at least 8 hours
2/3 cup cooked ham, diced small
1 large yellow onion, diced
4 cloves of garlic, minced
1 bunch of Italian parsley, chopped
2 tbsp brown sugar
2 tsp dried thyme
salt, black pepper and cayenne pepper, to taste

Preparation:

Add all of the ingredients to a stock pot with enough water to cover the ingredients by slightly more than 2". Bring to a boil, then reduce to medium low heat and simmer, covered, for about 4 hours, stirring occasionally. Remove from heat, season to taste with salt, black pepper and cayenne pepper and serve hot.

Swiss Chard and Kidney Beans

Number of servings: 4

Ingredients:

1 ½ cups cooked kidney beans (or 1 can, drained and rinsed if using canned beans)
1 large bunch of Swiss chard or rainbow chard, washed, patted dry and chopped roughly
1 tomato, diced
1 shallot, minced
2 cloves of garlic, minced
4 green onions, trimmed and sliced
2 tbsp olive oil
juice of ½ lemon
salt and black pepper, to taste

Preparation:

Heat the olive oil over medium heat in a large skillet (preferably a cast iron skillet). Once the oil is hot, add the garlic, shallot and green onions and cook for about 5 minutes, or until tender and fragrant, stirring occasionally. Add the kidney beans, diced tomato and chard and cover. Cook for 3 – 4 minutes or until the chard is just wilted. Add the lemon juice, stir well and cook for 1 more minute. Remove from heat, season to taste with salt and black pepper and serve at once.

Italian Zucchini Salad

Number of servings: 6

Ingredients:

2 large zucchini (or yellow crookneck squash – or one of each)
1 small red onion, minced
a few large basil leaves, chopped finely
¼ cup olive oil (use extra virgin olive oil for this recipe if you have it on hand)
3 tbsp pine nuts
2 tbsp coarsely ground salt (use 1 tbsp if you only have finely ground salt on hand)
juice of 1 lemon, or more to taste
salt, black pepper and crushed red pepper flakes, to taste

Preparation:

Heat a skillet over medium heat; do not add oil. Once the skillet is hot, add the pine nuts and cook for about 5 minutes or until lightly browned fragrant, stirring occasionally. Transfer to a small bowl and set aside.

Wash the zucchini or yellow squash and trim off the ends. Slice lengthwise into quarters and then into ½" thick slices. Transfer the sliced zucchini or yellow squash to a bowl and sprinkle with the salt, then toss to coat. Pour the salted squash into a colander in your sink and allow to drain for 30 – 40 minutes; the squash will soften during this time.

Rinse the squash very thoroughly under cold running water until most of the salt is removed. Pat dry and transfer to a mixing bowl. Add the remaining ingredients and stir well to combine, then season to taste with salt, black pepper and crushed red pepper flakes before serving.

Low GI Black Bean Dip

Number of servings: varies

Ingredients:

1 ½ cups refried black beans (homemade or 1 can premade)
1 cup salsa, your choice
1 cup plain lowfat yogurt
¼ cup shredded low fat sharp cheddar cheese
salt and black pepper, to taste

Preparation:

Preheat your oven to 325 F. Combine all of the ingredients except for the in a small, shallow baking dish. Sprinkle the bean mixture with the shredded cheese and bake for 15 minutes, or until the cheese is lightly melted and the beans are heated through.

White Bean Dip

Number of servings: varies

Ingredients:

3 cups cooked white beans (your choice) – or 2 cans, drained and rinsed
½ of a small red onion, minced
4 cloves of garlic, minced
½ cup chopped Italian parsley
¼ cup vegetable stock
2 tbsp olive oil (use extra virgin olive oil)
salt, black pepper and crushed red pepper flakes, to taste

Preparation:

Heat the olive oil in a saucepan; once the oil is hot, add the garlic and onion and cook until tender, stirring occasionally (about 3 – 4 minutes). Add the vegetable stock and beans and cook until heated through, then roughly mash with a potato masher. Add the parsley and mash a little more. Stir, season to taste with salt, black pepper and red pepper flakes, then stir again and remove from heat. Transfer the mixture to a bowl and refrigerate, covered, to chill. Serve cold or at room temperature.

Cucumber Salad

Number of servings: 4 – 6

Ingredients:

2 large cucumbers, peeled and sliced thinly
½ of a small onion, thinly sliced
3 cloves of garlic, crushed
1 cup white wine vinegar
1 tbsp sugar
2 tsp dill

Preparation:

Add the vinegar, crushed garlic, dill and vinegar to a bowl and whisk together until the sugar is dissolved and the garlic is well combined with the other ingredients. Add the cucumber slices to a bowl and pour the vinegar mixture over the cucumber and toss to coat. Cover and refrigerate for at least 2 hours and preferably overnight to allow the flavors to combine before serving.

Creamy Carrot Soup

Number of servings: 4

Ingredients:

1 lb carrots, scrubbed, trimmed and sliced
4 cups vegetable broth
1 small yellow onion, diced
1 sweet potato, scrubbed and diced small (peeling optional)
4 cloves of garlic, minced
½ of a bunch of cilantro, chopped
1 tbsp vegetable oil
salt and black pepper, to taste
4 tsp plain lowfat Greek yogurt, for serving

Preparation:

Heat the vegetable oil in a large saucepan over medium heat. Once the oil is hot, add the onion and garlic and cook until they're tender and start to brown slightly, about 5 minutes, stirring occasionally. Add the carrots and cook for another 5 minutes, stirring regularly, then add the vegetable broth and bring the mixture to a boil. Reduce the heat to medium – low and cover.

Simmer for 15 – 20 minutes or until the carrots are tender; the actual cooking time will depend largely on how thinly you slice the carrots. Remove from heat and transfer the soup to a blender or food processor along with the cilantro and blend until smooth; you'll probably need to puree the soup in two batches. Return the soup to the saucepan, season to taste with salt and black pepper and reheat. Divide among 4 soup bowls and serve hot, topped with 1 tsp of yogurt for each bowl.

Spinach Soup

Number of servings: 6

Ingredients:

2 (9 ounce) packages of spinach (wash and pat dry if you're not using prewashed spinach)
1 medium sized red onion, diced
1 large sweet potato, cubed (peeling optional)
2 Roma tomatoes, diced
2 cups watercress, washed, stems removed and chopped
6 cloves of garlic, crushed
3 cups vegetable broth
2 ounces shaved Romano cheese
¼ cup dry sherry (don't use cooking sherry)
1 tbsp butter
1 tsp oregano
1 tsp basil
salt and black pepper, to taste

Preparation:

Melt the butter in a large saucepan or stock pot over medium heat; add the garlic, onion, basil and oregano and cook until the onion and garlic are tender and begin to turn golden brown, about 5 minutes, stirring occasionally. Add the sherry and cook for 2 minutes to cook off the alcohol; add the sweet potato and vegetable broth. Bring the mixture to a boil and then reduce the heat to medium low. Cover the pot and simmer for 10 – 15 minutes, or until the sweet potato is tender.

Stir in the spinach and cook until just wilted, about 5 minutes. Transfer the soup to a blender or food processor and blend until smooth (you may need to do this in batches). Return the blended soup to the pot and cook until heated through. Remove from heat, stir in the watercress and diced tomato, season to taste with salt and black pepper and serve hot, topped with shaved Romano cheese.

Tomato – Basil Soup

Number of servings: 2

Ingredients:

3 large tomatoes, diced
3 Roma tomatoes, diced
1 small white onion, diced
6 large basil leaves, chopped
2 cloves of garlic, sliced
½ cup water
2 tsp olive oil
1 tsp white pepper
salt and black pepper, to taste

Preparation:

Heat the olive oil in a saucepan over medium heat. Add the onion, garlic, chopped basil and tomatoes until the onions soften. Add the white pepper, cover and reduce the heat to medium low. Simmer, covered, for 30 minutes and remove from heat. Transfer the soup to a food processor or blender and puree until smooth. Return the soup to the pan and cook until heated through. Season to taste with salt and black pepper and serve.

No-Crust Pumpkin Cheesecake

Number of servings: 8

Ingredients:

6 eggs
1 lb cream cheese, softened at room temperature
½ cup sugar free or reduced sugar maple syrup
1 ½ cups cooked pureed pumpkin (homemade or 1 can if using premade)
½ tsp Stevia or an equivalent amount of the sugar substitute of your choice
1 tsp cinnamon
½ tsp nutmeg
cooking spray

Preparation:

Start by preheating your oven to 350 F. Add all of the ingredients to a blender or food processor and puree until smooth and thoroughly combined. Lightly coat a pie dish with cooking spray and pour in the mixture. Bake for 50 minutes to 1 hour, or until the center is set. Remove from the oven and allow to cool to room temperature, then refrigerate and chill thoroughly before serving.

Zucchini Casserole

Number of servings: 8

Ingredients:

2 cups cooked zucchini, yellow crookneck squash or any other
summer squash you prefer
2 large eggs, beaten
1 cup whole wheat cracker crumbs or bread crumbs
1 cup milk
½ cup butter, softened at room temperature
2 tsp dried parsley
2 tsp dried chives
salt and black pepper, to taste
cooking spray

Preparation:

Preheat your oven to 375 F. Place the cooked squash into a large
bowl; mash roughly with a potato masher. Add the remainder of
the ingredients and stir well to combine. Lightly coat a 8 x 8
baking dish with cooking spray and bake for about 35 minutes or
until lightly browned on top. Remove from the oven and allow the
casserole to cool slightly before serving.

Baked Rutabega Fries

These baked rutabaga fries have a wonderful flavor which make them a nice change of pace from conventional potato fries – and they won't send your blood sugar levels on a roller coaster either!

Number of servings: 4

Ingredients:

1 rutabega, scrubbed and trimmed
1 clove of garlic, minced
1 tsp olive oil
1 tsp dried rosemary, minced
salt and black pepper, to taste

Preparation:

Start by preheating your oven to 400. Slice the rutabaga into thin (but not shoestring) fries and place in a bowl with the garlic, rosemary, olive oil and a little salt and black pepper. Toss to coat the rutabaga fries with the seasonings. Place the rutabaga fries on a baking sheet in a single layer, leaving room in between each fry. Bake for about 30 minutes or until they're crisp on the outside, turning once halfway through. Remove the fries from the oven, season to taste with salt and black pepper and serve hot.

Nakkileipa (Finnish style crispbread)

Number of servings: 12 pieces

Ingredients:

1 cup warm water
1 tbsp active dry yeast
2 cups rye flour
2/3 cup all purpose flour
1/3 cup pumpernickel flour, plus a little extra for flouring your work surface
1 ½ tsp salt

Preparation:

Add the warm water to a small bowl and sprinkle with the yeast; set aside while you mix together the dry ingredients in a large bowl. Once the yeast foams up (about 5 minutes), pour it into the dry ingredients and mix until a soft dough forms. Flour a clean work surface with pumpernickel flour, turn out the dough onto your prepared work surface and knead gently, adding the pumpernickel flour a little at a time. Shape the dough into a long roll, then cut it into twelfths, rolling each into a ball. Cover the dough with a clean kitchen towel and allow it to rise for 30 minutes.

While the dough is rising, preheat your oven to 425 F and lightly flour 2 large non stick baking sheets with pumpernickel flour. Roll out each ball of dough to a roughly 4" circle. Transfer the circles of dough to baking sheets and pierce each in several places with a fork. Bake the crispbread for about 10 minutes or until lightly browned. Remove from the oven and allow to cool completely on a wire rack before serving or storing for later use.

Polynesian-Style Ceviche

Number of servings: 4

Ingredients:

8 ounces of white fish filets (any kind you like), cut into bite sized pieces
1 medium sized red onion, diced
1 tbsp grated ginger
2 Thai chilies, minced (use more or less to taste)
juice and zest of 2 limes
salt and black pepper, to taste

Preparation:

Combine all of the ingredients except for the fish in a non-reactive (glass or ceramic) bowl. Add the fish and stir gently to combine. Add salt and black pepper to taste, cover the bowl and refrigerate for at least 1 hour – the fish will turn opaque and white when it's ready to eat, but an hour or two in the refrigerator will allow the flavors to combine. Leave covered in the refrigerator until ready to serve.

Cucumber – White Bean Salad

Number of servings: 6

Ingredients:

1 ½ cups cooked white beans (your choice) – or 1 can precooked
white beans, drained and rinsed
2 cucumbers, peeled and diced
4 Roma tomatoes, diced
¼ cup finely crumbled feta cheese
2 tbsp balsamic or red wine vinegar
2 tbsp water
1 tbsp tahini
juice of 1 lemon
1 tsp oregano
salt and black pepper, to taste

Preparation:

Add the cucumber, tomatoes and beans to a large salad bowl. Stir,
cover and refrigerate for 2 – 3 hours. When you're ready to serve
the salad, whisk together the vinegar, water, tahini, lemon juice,
oregano and season to taste with salt and black pepper. Add the
dressing and feta cheese to the salad and toss well to combine.

Breakfast

Whole Grain Blueberry Pancakes

Number of servings: 4

Ingredients:

1 cup whole wheat flour
1 large egg
¾ cup milk (or almond or soy milk, if desired)
½ cup fresh (or thawed frozen) blueberries
2 tsp artificial sweetener (your choice)
1 ½ tsp baking powder
a pinch of salt
cooking spray

Preparation:

Add the flour and baking powder to a small bowl and stir well to combine (you can also sift them together, if desired). In a separate bowl, whisk the milk, egg, salt and sweetener until slightly frothy. Add the dry ingredients until they're just moistened, then fold in the blueberries. Stir until there are no large lumps left (but not until smooth) and set aside.

Lightly coat a heavy skillet (preferably a cast iron skillet) and heat over medium heat. Once the skillet is hot, you're ready to start cooking the pancakes. Add about ¼ cup of batter per pancake (or more, if you'd like to make a smaller number of larger pancakes) and cook until bubbles stop forming and the bottom is golden brown. Flip and cook the other side until golden brown and transfer to a covered plate to keep warm until you're ready to serve the pancakes. Repeat the process until the batter is used up, then serve immediately.

Vegetable Frittata

Number of servings: 4 (4x ingredients)

Ingredients:

4 extra large eggs
½ cup green bell pepper, sliced into thin strips
1 clove garlic, minced
2 tbsp chopped Italian parsley
2 tbsp Romano or parmesan cheese, grated
2 tsp olive oil
juice of ½ lemon
salt and black pepper, to taste

Preparation:

Heat the olive oil in a skillet over medium heat. Once the oil is hot, add the sliced bell peppers, garlic and lemon juice and cook until tender. Season with a little salt and black pepper; remove from heat, but keep the burner going.

Beat the eggs together with the chopped parsley, parmesan and a little black pepper until combined, but do not overbeat. Return the skillet to the burner and pour the egg mixture over the peppers. Cook until the mixture is firm enough to flip, then turn over and cook for about 1 minute on the other side. Remove from heat and allow to rest for a minute or two before slicing and serving.

Tortilla de Patata y Espinacas (Spanish style potato and spinach omelet)

Number of servings: 8

Ingredients:

10 large eggs
14 ounces spinach leaves, washed (or use pre-washed spinach)
2 potatoes, scrubbed and sliced thinly
1 small red onion, sliced thinly
2 cloves of garlic, sliced thinly
1 tbsp olive oil
1 tsp oregano
a splash of milk
salt and black pepper, to taste

Preparation:

Place the spinach in a colander while you boil a pot of water. Once the water comes to a boil, pour it slowly over the spinach until it wilts; allow the spinach to drain.

Heat the olive oil in a large skillet over medium heat. Once the oil is hot, cook the potato and onion until the potato is soft, about 10 minutes, stirring occasionally. While the onion and potato cook, beat the eggs with the oregano and a little salt and black pepper; set aside.

Add the spinach to the skillet and stir to combine. Preheat your broiler. Pour the egg mixture into the skillet and cook until almost set. Transfer the skillet to the broiler and cook for about 2 minutes, or until the top is set.

Remove the skillet from the broiler and gently turn out the tortilla onto a large plate, then return to the pan and cook until both sides are finished. Return the tortilla to a plate and allow it to rest for 2 minutes before slicing and serving.

Dessert

Lemon Cake

This recipe is fairly high in sugar as low GI recipes go, so keep in mind that this lemon cake is meant only as an occasional treat and of course, only in sensible serving sizes.

Number of servings: 12 (2 small cakes)

Ingredients:

½ cup all purpose flour, sifted
¼ cup whole wheat flour, sifted
½ cup almond meal
½ cup powdered sugar
¼ cup butter, softened at room temperature, plus a little extra for greasing the cake pans
5 egg whites and 3 egg yolks
juice of 2 lemons
zest of 1 lemon
2 ½ tsp baking powder
½ tsp salt

Preparation:

Preheat your oven to 375 F. Cream the butter and sugar until smooth. Add the egg whites and whisk until the mixture becomes light and fluffy – the lighter this mixture is, the lighter and airier your cake will be. Add the lemon juice and zest, baking powder, flour, egg yolks and salt and mix until smooth.

Grease two small cake pans with butter and divide the matter between the prepared pans. Bake the lemon cakes for 15 – 20 minutes or until golden and sound hollow when the pans are tapped. Remove the cakes from the oven and allow them to cool completely on wire racks before slicing and serving.

Green Beans With Balsamic Glaze

Number of servings: 4

Ingredients:

2 cups green beans, trimmed and halved
2 cloves of garlic, sliced thinly
4 tsp of balsamic vinegar
2 tsp olive oil
salt and black pepper, to taste

½ cup water, for steaming

Preparation:

Add the green beans and water to a saucepan and steam for about 10 minutes, or until the green beans are crisp-tender. Drain and toss the green beans with the garlic, oil and vinegar. Return the pan to heat and cook until the vinegar is reduced to a glaze, stirring occasionally. Remove from heat, season to taste with salt and black pepper and serve.

Split Pea Soup

Number of servings: 4 as a main dish, 6 as a side dish

Ingredients:

1 ½ cups dry split peas
5 cups of chicken or vegetable stock
2 small onions, diced
2 small carrots, diced
4 cloves of garlic, minced
½ cup cubed ham
½ cup milk
1 tbsp olive oil
2 tsp thyme
1 bay leaf
salt and black pepper, to taste

Preparation:

Heat the olive oil in a very large saucepan or a stock pot over medium heat. Once the oil is hot, add the garlic, onion, carrots and ham and sauté until the onion turns translucent, 3 – 4 minutes, stirring occasionally. Add the remaining ingredients, bring the mixture to a boil and then reduce the heat to medium – low and cover. Simmer, covered, for 1 ½ hours, then add the milk and continue simmering until heated through. Remove the soup from heat, season to taste with salt and black pepper and serve hot.

Conclusion

The idea of going on a diet, especially something like a low glycemic index diet which you may not fully understand right away can be daunting. However, it doesn't have to be – and once you get started cooking low GI meals, you'll see that it can actually be quite easy, not to mention delicious.

Even if you're not used to eating whole grains and other healthier, lower GI foods, you'll soon find that it becomes second nature and that you'll make healthier choices on your own. In fact, many people find that after making the switch to a more nutritionally sound (not to mention healthier) diet, they lose their taste for the high GI, heavily processed foods they'd been used to eating before; hopefully, that will be your experience with our low GI recipes and you'll be not just ready, but eagerly looking forward to making low GI eating a new and healthier habit.

Printed in Poland
by Amazon Fulfillment
Poland Sp. z o.o., Wrocław

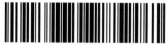